Mortality & Magic:
Facts & Fairytales for the Hereafter

Printed in USA by 48HrBooks (www.48HrBooks.com)

Cover Design Mastermind Graphics
info@mm-graphics.com

Mortality

&

Magic

Facts and fairytales
for the hereafter

Placid Bone
Illustrations by Eric Bloom

Deadication

To all those who might one day
possibly die.

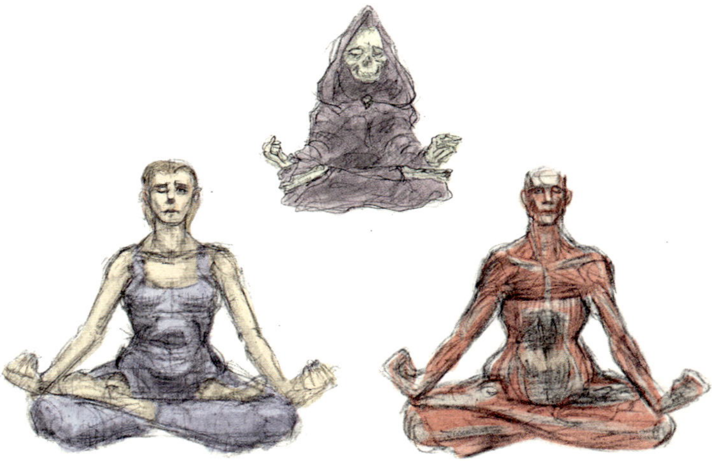

If one is capable of seeing
all the various endings,
in the end
there will be laughter.

-Hazrat Inayat Khan

FACTS

The origin of life:

Eighty-five percent of all human beings enter the planet through a vagina.

Fifteen percent of human beings arrive on Earth through another big gaping hole.

One hundred percent of all human beings will die.

There are three places to die.

There are four ways to die.

There are five stages of dying.

All of the material presented in this book on dying is factual.

Contents

Introduction
The most important day of your life

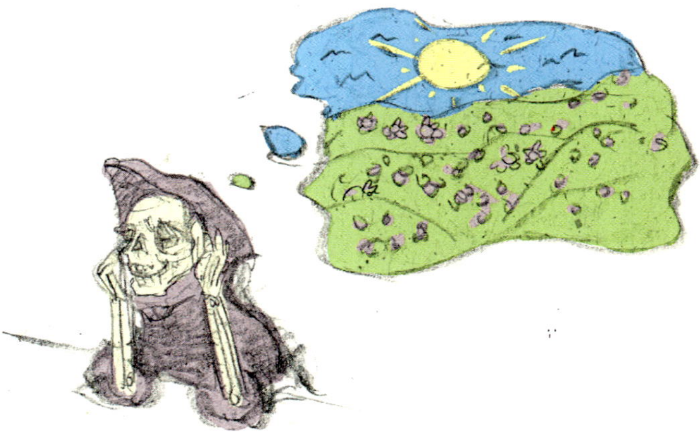

It is untrue that one's birth day marks the most important moment in a lifetime. Many of us get quite a few important days in our lives, some even more than 100. Each of us however, will have one and only one glorious day that will be our last.

If the weatherman predicts a 60% chance of rain and you so wisely pack an umbrella, then you have planned for the future. Why plan to arrive at work with dry clothes, and not plan for your last moments in the world? After all if you are 18 or 80 there is a 100% chance that one day you will permanently leave the planet Earth.

Dying can be planned. It can be envisioned like your graduation, your wedding or your birthday. If you could pass away in the most perfect way what would that look like? What would be the last music you hear - a live clarinet or a recorded Gregorian Chant? Would you want a religious passage or a touching Gibran poem read to you by a loved one? You have planned for the birth of your child, created nest eggs for future vacations, and rehearsed for countless ceremonies. You know how to plan, envision and inspire. Do the same for the finale of your life.

Medicine is sustained by one goal: to prolong life. Scientific advancements function only up to a certain point. The latest research remains at a loss to cure death, as such the personal mortality rate remains the same - one per person. I am

not promoting suicide. I am promoting healthy and happy living.

Dying is a stage of life. It is the last phase, and sooner or later we all reach there, even the unfortunate victims of sudden and immediate death will find themselves dying if only for a few seconds. You cannot die well unless you prepare for your passage. "What" you may ask, with the eager tone of a juvenile, "happens if I don't prepare for death?" Well, you still will die anyway. It's the difference between jumping out of plane with a parachute versus jumping out of plane without one. In both cases you land, but the preparation and forethought of a buffer makes all the difference.

Dying plans are for the healthy, chronically in-firmed, terminally ill and those who are just plain interested in life and healing. Similar to how a birth plan is as much for the father as it is for the mother, a plan for dying will inform not only those preparing to die but also their concerned caregivers. A plan for dying does not mean that we stop living. It is a recognition and a nod to Life that "Yes, I understand how this all ends and this is my final chapter." Decide the last pages of your autobiography. A complete life ends with a story that your loved ones will recount over and again.

A dying plan is no different than your drive through a fast food window…a little of "this", hold the "that", extra "this", plus a side of "that". It gives you a chance to figure out what is possible and what you would like. It refreshes the memories of your doctors and families during the process and ultimately gives you control. Your dying plan is a duty for the sake of the living. It is the answer to four questions that will quite literally change your life and all that remains of it.

This book is a "How to Die" guide promoting the good death. There are facts mixed with fairytales so you may understand through stories the journey to planning your last and most memorable party and date. The fairytales came about because everyone grows old except of course, our favorite childhood icons. Does Snow White have to remain forever 18? What if these legendary storybook characters did mature, and just as they taught us lessons for growing up they have more to teach us about growing old and dying. Sleeping Beauty taught us not to take food from strangers, yet she made us believe in true love. Now that she has been reunited with her Prince Charming what lessons about a peaceful passing can she share, having been there once before? What might a Dr. Seuss rhyme about dying teach children? Even Dorothy and her friends in Oz, as they grow old, can tell us new stories about finding home.

As you read each chapter the when, where, who, what, and how of your last days will begin to crystallize. You will then be ready to solve your personal immortal dilemma. Write down your answers. Share with your loved ones. Continue to live knowing that a foolproof even magical finale awaits you.

Chapter 1

Fact: Every day death is near

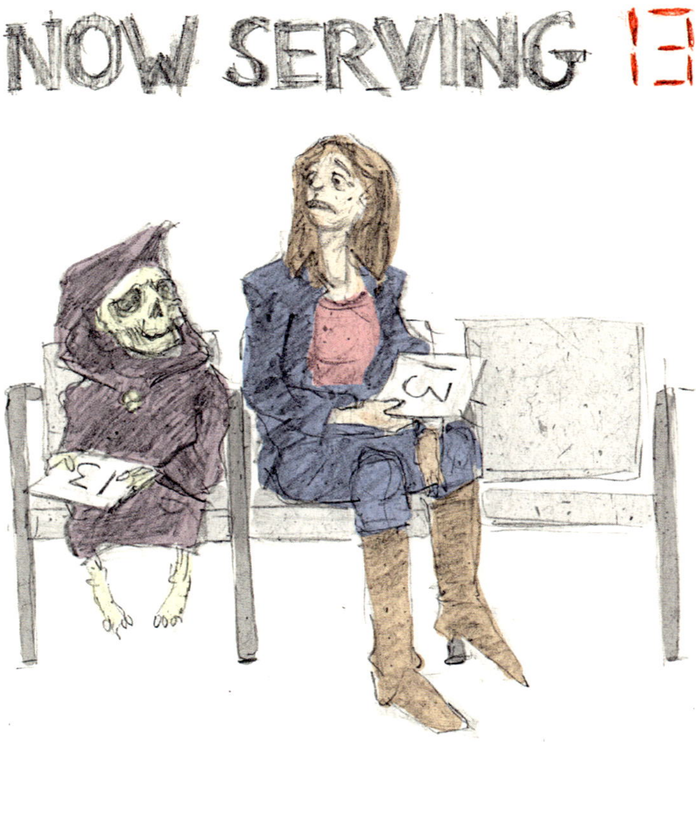

Going to the hospital is a lot like a trip to the circus. The doctors are the ring masters. Whirling around four-foot stethoscopes, stamping out disease, and taming death. The nurses are the concession stand sellers. Wearing the color of purity and cleanliness, they saunter through each room dispensing all modes of comfort providing stainless steel injections, white powders, and clear goo. Gofers scurry around offering a pair of socks, a tray of food, or a cup of water. Hospital administrators strut through the halls on stilts in black and white striped suits with ridiculously tall Abe Lincoln hats. Finally, send in the clowns. There must be clowns. The patients of every hue, costume and acrobatic ability. Over the loud speakers there is the constant refrain:

"Row, row, row your boat.
Gently down the stream.
Merrily, merrily, merrily, merrily
Life is but a dream."

Sometimes sung in a blues gospel tone, an operatic soprano, a rap, and a country music tune - all day long.

Painted on each wall is the mantra: Every Day Death is Near.

These were my thoughts as I ascended in the green elevators to the in-patient ward. This morning I was visiting the mother of Cornwall - my neighbor. His matriarch is affectionately known as

Cheechee. This was her third month in the hospital after a surgery had spiraled into one complication after another. Shuttling back and forth between the Intensive Care Unit (ICU) and the medical floor, this lady looked worn out. Today she was in the company of her son Cornwall. The other woman, his sister, who greeted me was petite Irene. She had the body of a prepubescent 14 year-old. Her 40-year struggle with alcohol came with the blessing of being currently unemployed and now the full-time warden over her mother's health.

My arrival had been announced as, "The doctor is coming!" My visit was partly as a familial obligation, a good Samaritan, and a researcher on mortality. I instinctively knew it would be in poor taste to approach Cheechee with a kiss followed by "How does it feel to be dying?" I smiled and observed instead. My comments were mostly to improve her comfort; Brush her hair. Cut and paint her nails. Massage her feet. Read to her. These were taken as strict medical advice and instructions were dispensed to the eight other children. "Bring homemade soup." Cornwall texted; followed by "Don't forget the hairbrush."

Cornwall and Irene enthusiastically attended to the task of massaging Cheechee's legs. The old woman perked up. She picked up her head to eye what was going on at the foot of the bed. A grin pierced through her perpetual frown. She still may pull through. Yet there was so much standing between her and the exit door of the hospital.

The paradox of hospitals is that they can make you sick. Cheechee was the victim of many well intentioned interventions and doctors. First there was the surgery to remove a cancer in her womb. The wound was healing then someone noticed feces oozing from the stitches in her belly.

Impossible! The pipes that carry stocl are closed until they exit through the anus. Everything is closed until it is opened by the well intentioned scalpel of an overzealous surgeon. The bowel was nicked creating a free passage into her wound and other organs. The treatment - plastic. Cheechee got lots of it. Plastic to cover the wound; plastic to suck out the stool; plastic in her stomach to feed her; and plastic in her neck to help her breathe when the plastic in her mouth could no longer remain in place. The most recent piece of plastic was an intravenous line that was removed from her right arm a few days earlier. The job of this intravenous line was to put water in Cheechee's veins but instead it gave saline to the tissue under the skin. Her right arm was red, hot, swollen, and painful. Classic battle signs of the body fighting off bacteria. More obstacles between her and the exit door to home.

It is a terrible experience that only few can understand. A healthy vibrant woman walks into a place fully expecting to go home in a day or so to a better life only to realize after the third month that she is lying in the same hospital bed. I imagine it's like boarding a fabulous cruise ship expecting to deport on some sunny paradise isle, only to wake up clinging to drift wood in the middle of the ocean. Day after day, wondering - "When and how will this end?" As the hours tick by, "When will I go home?" is asked with enthusiasm and even hope. After 30 days, despair takes over. "I just want out of here!" someone in the ocean screams. Hopelessness ensues after 60 days and three words beg for kindness, "Let. Me. Go."

I found Cheechee letting go of the driftwood and waiting to die. She was literally at the crossroads of life. Turn left to live longer. Turn right to die. Any day an overwhelming infection of the blood could steer her to the right and within days she would be gone. This truth was better left unsaid. Words hold power. Proof of this lies in the often overheard and instinctive command to a total stranger "Bless you!"

Even though she may have been dying, we were still taking care of her life. Today she needed to get out of bed and sit in a chair. No one should take for granted the ability to sit, stand, or walk. It is a luxury. On the list of biological requirements to sustain life, it is a want not a need. It is swiftly expendable. The maxim "use it or lose it" is epitomized in muscle and bone. After three moons of lying in bed, Cheechee's legs could not cope with the force of gravity. After bearing 10 children and 40 years of the great Western diet, old girl was 190 pounds of soft yielding dough. It took four of us, each attached to a limb, plus an automatic bed to prop her into a sitting position and allow her legs to dangle. For a full 2 minutes she sat there slumped over, eyes closed and moaning "Put me back. Please put me back."

Cornwall and Irene looked at me, both with furrowed brows and proceeded to ask a most peculiar question, "Is she going to die?"

I quickly role-played the various scenarios as to what my answer should sound like. If I were a preacher, an emphatic "Yes of course, we all are going to die!" A stockbroker might have said, "There's a 50/50 chance. Best to place your money on the affirmative." A lawyer would have grinned and reassured them "No, of course not. I guarantee it."

When is the best time to discuss dying? Cheechee was knocking on death's door. Now is the time. For Cornwall it might be last month when he was in the emergency department flirting with the doctor who was sewing up his foolish embrace with a box cutter. For Irene it might be during her Friday pedicures. Like the fortune in the cookie, it is different for everybody, often obscure and requires context. Confucius say: Eat, drink and be merry. Imhotep say: Eat, drink and be merry, for tomorrow we die.

Chapter 2
THE WHEN

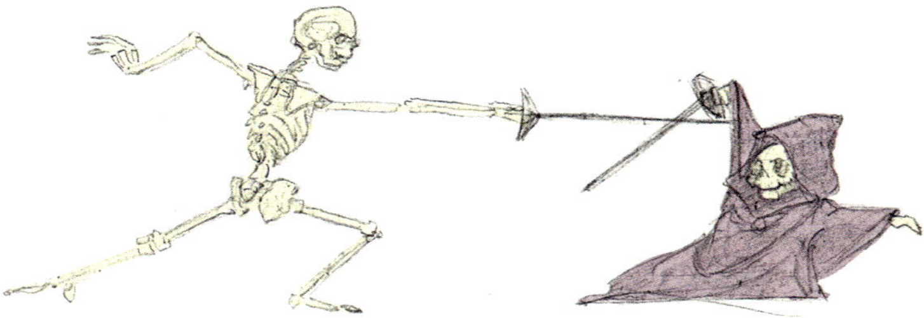

Fact:
Not if but when

Before is always different from after. A fact mother nature has made astoundingly apparent during the hours that each human is born, and when each one dies. Being dead is very different from dying. Most people can tell when someone is dead - the no-pulse, no-breathing, and stiff-as-a-board thing is hard to fake. Akin to watching a baby exiting the birth canal versus greeting the baby after the umbilical cord has been cut and the baby has been wiped clean from the amniotic slop; birthing is different from being alive as dying is as different from being dead.

As a Board Certified Emergency Medical Doctor I have witnessed hundreds of people dying, most of them without a plan. This is not a slight on my medical expertise, but a testament that everyday death is near, especially so in the emergency department. For the 56 year-old accident victim, dying came as a complete surprise to everyone including himself. As I cared for this man and other dying patients, I am reminded of a quote from the great King Yudhisthira. When asked, "What is the most wonderful thing?" He replied, "Hundreds and thousands of living entities meet death at every moment. Still, those who remain aspire for a permanent situation here. What could be more amazing than this?"

I understood my mission: Teach humans how to die well. Dying has a beginning, middle, and end. The beginning starts with the acceptance of death as a natural progression of things to come. Many of us will not know when death will come. Only death by corporal punishment (aka torture, an extreme form of capital punishment) or successful suicide comes with the advantage of a specific date and time. Doctors will never be this precise. The question of when do you want to die at first appears unanswerable - even absurd.

Eastern practitioners, spiritual leaders, and most importantly patients, all agree that thoughts create and mold the future. In Eastern medicine, thoughts are known to be discrete packets of energy that go forward and do what they were intended for, meaning that if the thought of the thinker was: "Today is going to be great day!" then this good-day-thought is now released into the atmosphere to create, you guessed it, "a good day." Western medicine refers to this same concept as the "Placebo Effect" which is another way of saying we can't measure it, we can't see it, we sure as hell can't prescribe it, but it works. And it does work. If you think that your cancer will kill you in 30 days, then it probably will. But, if you believe that you will live to 100, you are more likely to survive very close to that number. Unless, for some reason, death decides otherwise.

People have stayed their dying to finish one last task or to say one last goodbye. One sickly woman, determined to take her last breath in her birth land of Uruguay, did not want to burden her son with the bureaucracy of transporting her body between countries. She boarded the plane to her birth place and for the next week reunited with old friends and family of long ago, then quietly laid down on her bed and calmly passed away, alone.

If age is just a number then believe the age you die is a choice. Commit to an age, right now, that you expect to live until. Write it down. Be convinced. You have nothing but time to lose.

Fairytale:
Wolf & Little Red
(the acceptance of dying)

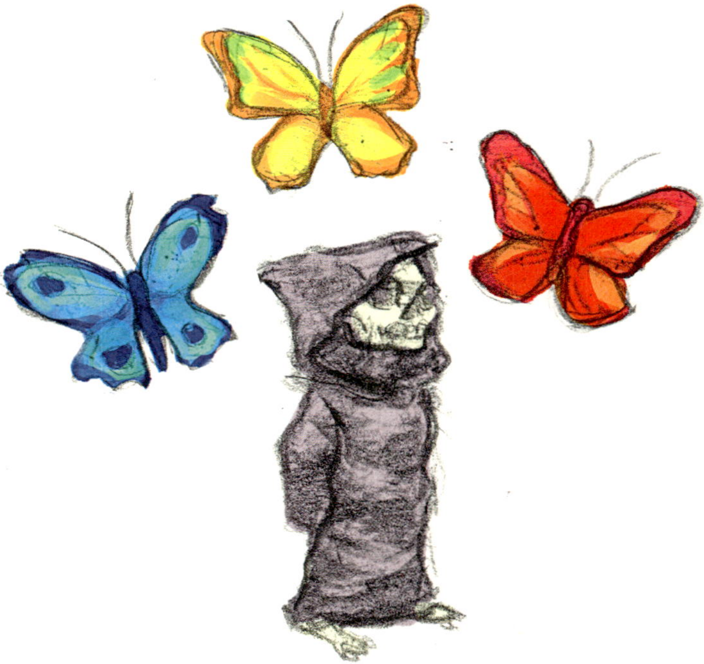

My name is Wolf, as in big and bad. I have some news. Your grandmother is dead.

Red stood still and blinked her eyes forcefully. "Dead" was not a word she knew the exact meaning of, only that it was an important four letter word, along with damn and shit. Two words she often heard as her parents were going through a divorce. Red needed to exit the daily screaming match, that was her short but wide 12 year-old life, and Granny needed winter provisions.

The assignment was simple and mutually beneficial, a weekend visit to Grandma's house. After a mixture of apples, zucchini, and fresh herbs were tightly packed into a weaved basket and the requisite red hood was donned, the girl was on her way. Don't talk to strangers was her mother's final mandate.

Up the hill and past the lake, out pops a talking Wolf. Strange at first, but the young female has not lived enough to know the art of disguise. After the Wolf delivers the matter of fact message about Granny's demise, Red, remembering her mother's words, is faced with only one decision either turn back or move forward.

What happens next proves that even a child knows the value of silence as evidenced by the natural order of developmental milestones, first hearing then speech. Understanding comes before language. Adults should never forget this simple fact, Red thinks, it could save marriages even countries. Each being fixed for the same reason - the children. Red brings her thoughts back to the present moment as she remains still and listens.

I wanted to make sure you knew. It was not my fault, offered the Wolf.

Until then, Red didn't know that death could be blamed on someone. She thought it was like an itch or a sneeze. A thing that just happened. Quickly her pre-teen brain blurted out; How do you know?

Thus started a much longer tale, dear reader, about how exactly the big bad Wolf found himself at Grandma's house on the very day she died. Some of you will remember from younger days that while his motives were less than kindhearted, you will swear with vehement affirmation that the wolf never killed Grandma, he only stuffed her in the closet while others who no longer recall the ending of common folk stories will remain unsure. The Wolf's alibi as to his whereabouts are sound. The details will only be recalled to make a specific point, that this fairytale is not about murder, but another sinister tool to teach a child about the end of life.

The Wolf finishes his rather lengthy defense - And that's how I found her, stiff and mottled. Are you scared? Sad?

Uhh. Uhh. Red wags her head no. We are all going to die. All of us get there sooner or later. Haven't you heard about the Caterpillar? My mom read me a story about a caterpillar that morphs into a butterfly, expecting me to believe it is a lesson of change, but it's about dying. The caterpillar lives a short 7 days, then dies. While he is dying, he wraps a cocoon around himself and these imago cells breakdown his body into goo and then a slow rearrangement starts. If our lives are anything like the caterpillar's, then I am not scared. What an upgrade for the caterpillar. First hairy and slow, now beautiful and winged.

CHAPTER 3
The What

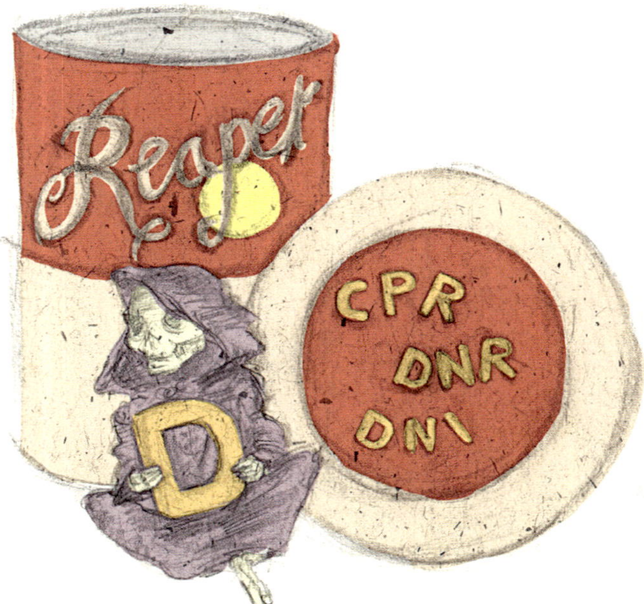

Fact:
CPR will not save you
(like in the movies)

Perhaps you find yourself or your loved one with diabetes, heart failure, cancer, or in some cases all three. You are going to die. No need to feel special because the rest of us are too. The image of a dying white-haired grandmother lying in bed surrounded by her children with one IV bag hanging by her bedside is familiar. The nurse solemnly comes to give her a morphine injection. The grandmother's eyes close. Her grip slackens and her breathing ceases. Finally, the soft weeping of family members. This is what most of us want for our loved ones and ourselves. Television would have us believe that this happens to everyone. Not so in any hospital or emergency department in the country. Technology has made dying a very noisy affair. There are bells and dings of machines coupled with the chatter of patients and staff squeezed into small spaces, add to that the occasional satanic screams of a nearby schizophrenic or drunk patient being physically restrained. If you want the television version of death, stay at home to chant or pray with your dying family member. Whisper your apologies and goodbyes.

For many of us, the last leap into the hereafter for the unprepared is scripted into predictable stages. A significant few will succumb to instantaneous oblivion as they crash in a plane, tongue kiss the steering wheel in an unseat-belted Porsche, or find themselves on the greeting end of a bullet. Trauma is still one of the top five faces of death in Western nations or infectious disease in the developing world. But much disease come from the droves of innocent lives that act literally on the advice of the Budweiser commercials and drown their liver and kidneys in alcohol. Or young girls who believe in the sexiness of sucking on sticks of cigarettes and end up with lung, lip, or laryngeal cancer. Or little kids orphaned off to corporate foster homes of Nintendo and Cartoon network so that the only thing that develops is their waistline. In Western countries most of us will die from a chronic disease such as coronary artery disease, hypertension, cancer, or diabetes.

The last hours of your life will pass in one of two ways, the planned or the unplanned death. The difference between the two is the answer to one simple question. Do you want to be in the category of "Do Not Resuscitate (DNR) and Do Not Intubate (DNI)?" The terms DNR, DNI are used frequently in the medical field and need to be understood by everyone. The term DNR communicates to your physician that if your heart were to stop pumping, that is, if you were to die, would you want to be resuscitated? Resuscitation is usually explained to the patient in polite terms like cardiopulmonary resuscitation (CPR), defibrillation, and injectable drugs. For many of you who have taken a CPR class, memories of gently thrusting on a dummy's chest and blowing air into its mouth will resurface. DNI is also explained to patients in heroic medical speak, "If you can no longer breathe on your own, we will put you on a breathing machine that will breathe for you." What actually happens in a code blue situation, is usually pre-hospital providers find you at home after you have collapsed. They check for a pulse and find none. Then they shock your chest with electricity, push on your chest to pump your heart from the outside often times breaking your ribs and injecting drugs like epinephrine, also known as adrenaline into your veins to jump-start your heart. Around the same time they put a breathing tube about 9 mm in diameter into your mouth to your lungs (a typical straw is about 3 mm in diameter) and hook you up to a machine that will thrust air into your lungs.

As a patient, you are forced to answer both questions. What do you want your doctor to do if your heart stops beating or your lungs were to stop breathing? You could answer yes to one and no to the other. Yes, I want my heart resuscitated, but no, I do not want to be hooked up to a breathing machine. From a doctor's point of view this is nonsense. One cannot have a working heart and lungs that do not inflate. Vice versa, one cannot have lungs that breathe but a heart which does not pump. The function of the heart and lungs are married from birth. Until death do they part.

During the 1950's CPR was created and implemented. For a healthy soldier in their 20's and 30's who gets shot or is in a car crash, CPR has been shown to be effective. Even for the person in their 50's and 60's that suddenly drops dead, the odds are high that they have had a massive heart attack which caused the electricity in their heart to have a chaotic surge. CPR and defibrillation have been shown to be extremely beneficial. This is why there are now defibrillators in airports, stadiums and other public places. CPR was never designed for the 70, 80, or 90 year-old with multiple medical problems. The success rate is quite small.

The real tragedy is that the medical profession offers one a false choice. Do you want to be resuscitated is a horrible way to phrase a question regarding your life. An answer of "No, I do not want to be resuscitated" seems to imply that nothing will be done to help you when you're dying. The dying person can still receive pain medication, antibiotics, and breathing assistance that is not invasive. Comfort will still be provided by the medical staff. Indeed, it must be the most important goal of the medical encounter.

The real question that you need to answer for yourself is, "When is it okay for me to die?" You can only answer this question if you have thought and planned your death. The question we doctors need to pose to our patients even if we have just met them a few minutes prior in the emergency department is, "Are you prepared to die today?"

If you are a robust 50 year-old, then the answer may justifiable be "Not today!" Even for a tough 90 year-old the answer may also be "No!" However, if you are a 60 year-old with one leg amputated, with a kidney transplant and no quality of life, then you may well decide that for you to die today would be just fine. Perhaps you hold the view that there is no such thing as untimely death, so whatever day you die then so be it.

The best decisions are informed decisions. What doctors do not communicate well is that even if you choose "to have everything done" meaning that you are not in the category of DNR or DNI, there is a good chance that you will die anyway. Statistically, the older you are and the more disease you have, the more likely that today will be your last day and that CPR will not be effective. Some would argue "Try any way - what have I got to lose if I am going to die either way?"

Instead of strangers witnessing blood and vomit come from your mouth as the breathing tube is placed, you could have your favorite verse whispered to you repeatedly by a loved one. These are not trivial matters. They will help you have the perfect death and provide unspeakable comfort to your grieving loved ones. Thankfully the term Allow Natural Death (AND) is slowly replacing the outdated and poorly worded question of DNR or DNI. By choosing AND, you are telling your medical providers that when my heart stops or when my breathing, stops please allow me to die. The acronym AND is suggestive of the original old english meaning of "and" which is "thereupon or next" suggesting that more will happen. Other things are to come.

While your last wishes may be to pass on among the tranquility of your loved ones, the Emergency Medical Service (EMS) cannot simply take the word of your well meaning family members. If in a panic, a family member accidentally calls 911 because you have collapsed and they are not sure why, EMS arrives and confirms that you are dead, meaning you have no pulse and you are not breathing, they are obligated to initiate CPR. You will not be able to hear your wife hum your favorite lullaby, if specific documents signed by you, the patient, and notarized for that particular state cannot be provided. This fact was sadly illustrated to me one day at work when two octogenarians arrived within one hour of each other - Mrs. Jones from a rehab center and Mr. Jones from a private home. The two patients came to the emergency department after suddenly collapsing in front of people who knew their wishes were to be in the DNR/DNI category. No paperwork meant that our EMS providers were forced to press, stick, stuff and shock these two people for over one hour even though the chance of meaningful survival is less than 1%. This behavior underscores the fact that at 87 years old it is okay to die.

Dying in this new millennium presents two problems and only two. The first is we will be waiting to die. Waiting is something many of us do not enjoy. Longevity, in some circles, is synonymous with prolonged dying. The ideal situation is to go to sleep and wake up dead. No pain, no theatrics - a simple slipping away into the dark of night. Odds are you will probably not be among the lucky few that death arrives this way. As nursing homes become holding cells for people ailing from dementia, stroke, frailty or AIDS, dying has become highly medicalized. All this waiting, of course, gives you more time to discuss and decide your immortal dilemma.

The second problem of dying in the 21st century is not having a plan. Your great-grandfather never had to worry about whether he was going to lose his memory and be labeled as having Alzheimers, when Gin and Tonic were perfectly willing to take the blame. Dying from dementia often means becoming a stranger to your loved ones and an unintended burden to them. While syphilis, not AIDS, was the sexually transmitted disease in vogue during your grandmother's time, no one suspected her late night trips to the neighbor's house was anything but altruism in an apple pie. Dying with AIDS has been judged by some as a shameful death. One that leaves the dying person even more isolated. Burdensome and shameful are not descriptions of the good death. One should plan an artful passing. For the sanity of your loved ones, do not leave it up to them to answer your immortal dilemma.

Fairytale:
A Conversation with Pinocchio, Dr. Frank & Beauty

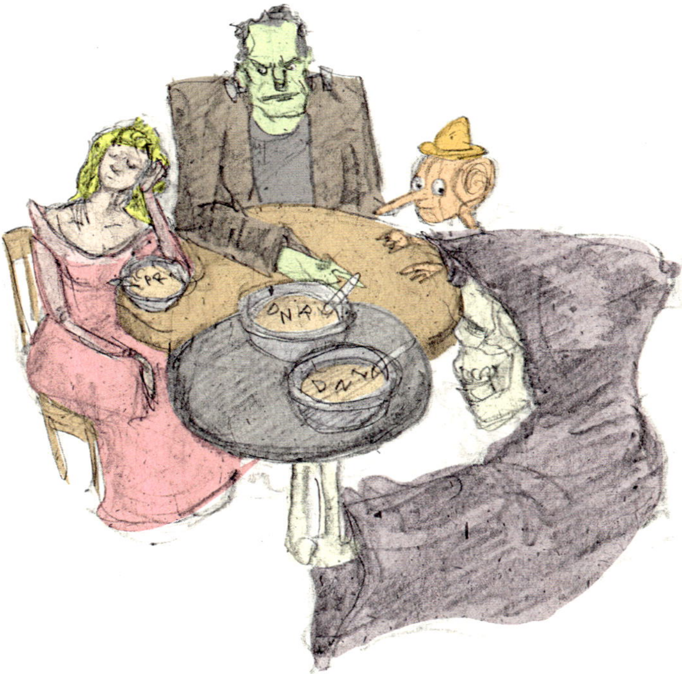

Pinocchio, Frankenstein, and Sleeping Beauty are three virtuosos on dying. Pinocchio wished to be a real boy for a long time. He knows what it is like to cling to the idea of life while not being alive. Frankenstein is a monster made of various dead body parts. He used to have a serious chip on his shoulder but after intensive counseling and 7 years in the English as a Second Language Program, he is now a physician. He is also a master on how medical terms such as CPR, DNR, and DNI actually translate into medical practice. Sleeping Beauty was asleep for more than 100 years. She knows dead. She knows alive.

The three wise ones are seated for lunch. Having achieved a certain level of notoriety throughout their lives, each feel that they are The Expert on the topic of dying.

After lying in slumber for over 100 years, Sleeping Beauty believes she knows firsthand exactly what it means to be dead. What was her last vivid memory? An unforgettable trek through the woods. "It was a sunny day," she recalled. "The air wus crisp. The birds wus chirpin'. I went to pick roses for Mamaw. When the thorn pricked my finger, I thought nuthin' of it. Then when I reached home I felt faint. I remember layin' my head down in Mamaw's lap. And that was awl she wrote." The southern belle threw her hands up in the air in an exasperated motion. "My po' muscles just wasted away till I was nuttin' but skin and bones. Skin got so pale I looked damn near like life wusn't in me. Until, well you know the rest: the kiss that brought me back and my prince CHARMing." Her drawl stretched her beloved's name out long and wide. "Havin' died once, I cherish everythin' about life. If they ask me if I want my heart started by electricity or if I want my lungs hooked up to a machine, I have one word for them - Hellsyeah!" Her hands akimbo, shot to her hips as if striking a pose for a Vogue Magazine. "Resuscitate my fine behind!"

"Vait! Vait! Beauty," interjected Frankenstein. His lispy German accent still prominent even after years of living abroad. "Cardiopulmonary resuscitation doesn't verk for everyone!" The narcoleptic Sleeping Beauty begins to nod off to sleep with her head propped up by her left hand. Frankenstein violently pounds the table. The green monster lets a rusty smile creak onto his face as he assures his startled friend, "You are young and healthy. CPR was designed specifically for people like you." Embarrassed by the sudden interference of deep sleep, Beauty with eyes half closed shines her pearlies back at him. "Yeah, yeah, Frankie Baby. I am the poster child for CPR. Who wudun't wanna bring ME back if I suddenly died?"

Frankenstein lets his eyes rest on her exposed and healthy bosom, "During var time CPR was for soldiers whose heart and lungs failed. It may even verk for the healthy 70 year-old." Beauty smiles drunkenly as her head gives way to a sudden bobble.

"But Beauty, fast forward to 30 years from now when you are in your 90's, CPR most likely won't verk." Frankenstein wonders if she is wearing a black or red bra. "This may come as a surprise, but the older you are the more likely that today you might be dead." After a long pause,

"It's a joke!" Frankenstein laughs maniacally, throwing his head back.

"For me," Frankenstein continues, "I have the vords DNR/DNI tattooed on my chest." He opens his shirt flashing his green skin at the other two. Sure enough in bold letters stretching from the right to left nipple are the words: DO NOT RESUSCITATE DO NOT INTUBATE. Pinocchio and Sleeping Beauty exchange a quizzical stare.

Ignoring them, Frankenstein continues his lecture, "After medical school, I know how frequently CPR is unsuccessful, even cruel. Someone pushes on your chest to mimic the verk of your heart from the outside. There is the crunching noise as your ribs are cracked." Sleeping Beauty frowns, "Dat sounds simply awful."

"Then a tube" Frankenstein curls his fingers to signal a big green - O. "Like a really big straw is pushed into your mouth. It is hooked up to a machine that thrusts air into your lungs." Frankenstein imagines giving Beauty mouth-to-mouth assistance. Beauty adds, "It sounds like it shewd work on anybody."

"Dah!, When your body is frail even these machines can't keep you alive." He places his hand over Beauty's hand, wishing they were alone. "Vat's verse is they may keep your heart pumping and your lungs inflated, but are you really alive?" He mimics a fading echo. "Alive? ALIVE?"

Pinocchio finally has something to say. "That is the most important question. What does it mean to be alive? For Sleeping Beauty who was resuscitated after being basically dead for a long time. Being alive for her is anytime her heart is beating."

"Bless your heart, sugar" Beauty interjects, "Being resuscitated ain't as simple as a smack on the lips. It means to bring back to life?"

Pinocchio continues "If you were a plant I would water you, change your soil, and put you in the sunlight. That would be me resuscitating you." Pinocchio smiles, proud of his ability to clarify the situation.

"We awl want life." Beauty adds with her southern twang.

"Dah," snorts Frankenstein "but CPR doesn't guarantee life. It means there will be pushing, shocking, and stuffing." His hands gesturing wildly. "In the end you may die anyway."

"So Frankie, what if I decide no to CPR like you described? That I don't want to be resuscitated." Pinocchio's voice is soft. "Will you, Dr. F. K. Stein, step over my dying body and leave me to suffer?"

"Nien, Pinocchio." Frankenstein wags a long green finger in his direction. "There is so much that can be done to help the dying person."

"If I were going to compose a question about what to do if you were on the verge of dying, it would be something like this" Frankenstein leans in close as if really talking to a patient "You are very sick. If your heart were to stop, do you vant nature to take its course? Do you vant God to decide? Or do you vant us to push on your chest and maybe break your ribs? Understand that if your ribs are broken, you vill need to be put on a breathing machine." He pauses dramatically. "You may never get off of the machine. More importantly you will not be able to say farewell to your loved ones. Vat do you Vant?"

"No bye-byes." Sleeping Beauty gasps, "Not again."

"Nothing is more painful to the human mind. If you vant to say goodbye then don't get on the breathing machine. This will allow you a good death." Frankenstein concludes.

"A good death!" squeals Pinocchio, "Is that like when Dr. Frankenstein took all those body parts and created you Frankie? A good death for them. A good life for you. Or when Beauty here fell off silently into a century slumber from a wicked witch's curse? Is that a good death? Or when Guiseppe died at home? The fairy angel came dressed in a black velvet dress with purple wings and sang a medley of Michael Jackson's tunes." Pinocchio begins the moonwalk across the table.

"Nien Pinocchio, a good death is a planned death." Dr. Frank grabs Pinocchio's ankle with his one finger forcing him to stop dancing and beams his green eyes intensely. "You have answered yes to the question. Is today a good day for me to die?"

Beauty says "Jus one minute, a good death for me would be kinda like the first time. I wanna go to sleep and wake up

DE...AD." She utters the word in two syllables. "How do I make this happen the second time around?"

Frankenstein responds matter of fact, "This is America, Beauty. Anything of importance is written down. If you suddenly collapse even as an octogenarian, the doctors will be forced to press, stick, stuff, and shock you."

Pinocchio chimes in "So it's okay to die at 80 years old?"

"Oh I've told you twiced Pinocchio, don't get fixed on a numbah! You can be dumber than a box of rocks," Beauty snorts, "some people at 80 are not a day over 60. Cum moi!" She presses an open palm against her chest. "While others are centurions. Or is it centenarians?"

Frankenstein interjects, "Zee point is, CPR is not a treatment for the dying process. Ven there is health, resuscitate. At the end of a chronic illness, it is inappropriate to revive. To give and receive words should be maintained through all stages of life."

Pinocchio stands up and puffs out his chest, superhero style, "If I have no signs of life. When I have no breath, no pulse. Then please, allow me a natural death."

Chapter 4
THE HOW

Fact:

There are four ways to die

Do you recall the time you spent going through puberty? The bodily changes were predictable with a start and a finish. Dying is no different. Experts in end-of-life care categorize dying into four groups. People will die of either sudden death, terminal illness, organ failure, or my favorite, good old fashioned frailty.

Although the focus of Western medicine is on prolonging life, it is possible and necessary to define when dying has begun for patients and the benefit of caregivers. Doctors can offer a calculation of weeks to months. If the doctor is wrong, you get to live another day or less. If you have a terminal illness and live in constant pain so that even breathing hurts, this may not be good news. You may be grateful for one more day to spend time with someone special.

"Wait Dr. DoGood," you demand while resisting the urge to roll your eyes, "which category do I fit into? I am not terminally ill, I don't have any diseases like diabetes or hypertension and I am only 42, so frailty for me is many decades away." To which the doctor hastily replies, "All of us are in the sudden death category until we are not." The best way to remove yourself from this category is to wear your seatbelt, avoid firearm usage and get regular medical checkups especially if an immediate family member has died suddenly.

Another way to not die suddenly is to develop a chronic disease through a lifestyle of excess. If death does not swipe you away from a massive heart attack, then overeating, drinking too much and smoking will probably result in a chronic disease. All chronic illnesses over time lead to organ failure. In Western countries, the organs that fail most commonly are lungs, liver, kidneys, and the heart. Aside from a transplant no cures exist as of today. There are medicines and machines that will temporarily, for several decades, perform the function of your failed organs. Patients either forget to take the medicine or get tired of using the machines accelerating the failure of these organs.

In heart failure, a patient unable to breathe rushes to the hospital. These visits become more frequent. Initially once a year then every six months, until you are hospitalized every month. Your family no longer dashes to the hospital with concern and fright because now you are there every week. They see it as just like the last time. Until you are dead, this visit to the hospital seems like every other time. You fully expect to go home. Weekly visits to the hospital because of organ failure indicate that dying has begun. You have six weeks to six months left to live.

Dying from terminal illness has been well studied. Perhaps through no fault of your own, you picked the short straw in the gamble of genetics. You discover a lump in your breast that you ignore as impossible to be cancer, given your youthful age of 29. By the time you see a doctor, the news is not good. The tumor is now squatting in your lungs and colon. Your illness is terminal after failed chemotherapy and radiation. You have less than one year remaining to live.

Frailty is your first year of life in reverse. When you were a baby you went from lying on your back to rolling over, sitting up, standing and walking, all within 12 months. People dying from frailty are often non-ambulatory and completely bed bound. Which sounds so damning, until you remember that so was every baby for their first six months. Within a year, a baby goes from being able to see only a distance of 3 feet to awareness of a medley of colors, sounds and shapes. Interviews with caregivers reveal that during the last year of life many elderly and frail persons do not recognize the faces of even close relatives. The final contrast between a blossoming baby and a withering frail person is language. As a baby you went from crying to cooing to babbling to your first words during your first year of life. If you are in the category of frailty, whether from dementia or a stroke in your last year of life, your speech will slow down and often times become a nonsensical gibberish. In the words of the famous Bob Marley "Once a man and twice a child. And everything is just for awhile."

Included in this last category of dying is the ability to sense that death is close. There are countless stories of yogis who knew death was approaching. The Buddha at the age of 80 knew his death was imminent. Call it intuition, spiritual advancement, or just plain luck. He gathered his followers. They cleared a space for him on the ground and he simply laid down on his right side and exhaled his last breath. I am certain, as Eastern philosophy teaches, this can be learned by anyone. Through proper breathing and meditation, one can know with certainty that one's last moments are near.

A trajectory is a path. Like a map it gives direction and length of time from point A to point B. A dying trajectory gives you an idea of the terrain ahead to traverse. Death from terminal illness is narrow with rocky hills. Death from organ failure is filled with long stretches of open highway and swooping valleys. Death from frailty is across bridges and through tunnels each time emerging with less than you began - fewer words, decreased awareness of your surroundings, and diminished ability to walk and stand. Frailty is in many ways a returning to the womb.

Here are some clues that you are dying: Are you visiting the emergency department more frequently because you cannot breathe because your lungs and heart are failing? Are you coming down with pneumonia or infections of the urinary tract because your immune system is weakening? Is your family considering placing you in a nursing home because you keep falling and have increased confusion? If you answered yes to any of these questions, death is approaching.

You may feel sad. But also feel relieved. Everyone knows what is happening. Your family may have a difficult time accepting that dying has begun. They feel that acceptance of death is giving up on living. Knowing that you will die next year puts into perspective that impending foreclosure. While finding out that you have only two weeks left to live may force you to reconcile sooner with your surly relative. If you had one day to live you would choose your words carefully. A glass of water would bring intense pleasure. There is power in information. Dialogue about when dying has begun will help you and your family prepare for your departure. In traditional Tibetan households, the doctor is called in at the time of death and whispers gently into the dying person's ear, "You're dying. It's ok. Let go."

Fairytale:
On the Yellow Brick Road -
trajectories of death

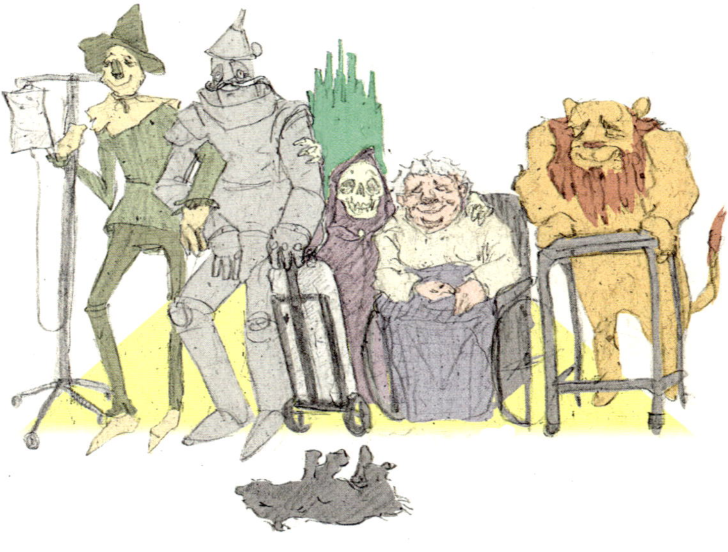

In the Land of Oz, the Lion did many great things with the courage given to him by the Wizard. He built. He defended. He invented. He made a family. As he grew old so did his heart. He lived every day as if it were his last. Ten days ago he was right, it was his last day. It happened suddenly. A slight twinge of pain in his left breast then a sheering ache in his heart and left arm all at once. Off he went, down the rabbit hole.

The Tin Man gave me the news when I visited him in the hospital. Tin was rushed to the emergency department again last night, unable to breathe. Three years prior he received a heart transplant. Apparently the one from the Wizard lasted only 20 years. Tin was having trouble breathing from his failing heart. He used to be home for a full six months before his next hospital stay, but lately he was in the hospital every other week. I asked him if he was sad that no one came to visit him this time. He shrugged his shoulders...What for? This time is just like the last time.

I sternly retorted: Until you are dead, Mr. Tin Man, your last visit to the hospital seems like every other time. Each time you fully expect to go home. Machines may keep your lungs working for another few years. But dying from a failing heart, weak kidneys, or exhausted lungs is a bit like an endless game of peeka-boo with death. Outside your hospital room stands the grim reaper with pink lipstick and a matching pink sickle. From the corridor you hear her husky sing-songy voice...*Wheeerrre are you*?

There you lay in bed, cowering under your sheets, huffing and puffing trying not to be found. This morning you thought - *She found me. This is it.* After a few hours the medicine kicks in, the breathing machine works harder. Poof. You can breathe easier. One more day to live for you Old Chap. My best approximation is that you have 6 weeks to 6 months left to live. One day the game will be over. His joints creaked loudly. He and his wheelchair rolled out of the hospital room in silence.

Death is Life's answer to "What to do with a fool?" It is Life's insurance policy. Otherwise some idiot might come along and wipe out existence for everyone. Before the birth of the first fool, human beings lived forever. As there was no quick and certain way to tell the difference between a fool and a wise person, it was easier and not to mention just plain fair for Life to invent Death for everyone.

At the funeral for the Lion, Dorothy struggled through *Somewhere Over the Rainbow*. She was not well herself. Dorothy was diagnosed with throat cancer and had just finished her third round of chemotherapy. Her voice was now raspy, reduced at times to a whisper. She fumbled a few lines, the most awkward being "If happy little blue birds *die* then why can't I?" The munchkins solemnly applauded.

The Scarecrow was also at the funeral. He was bolstered up by a cane and cast. The week prior he had fallen and broken his left hip. His straw pieces were scattered everywhere. He hasn't danced since. He was overheard telling Dorothy, "I am *SOO OVER* the rainbow."

There are four ways to die. Choose one. All of us, like Lion, are in the sudden death category. That is, you can always die suddenly. Until you don't. She may not agree with me, but Dorothy, has chosen to die from cancer. She could have chosen to die like the Tin Man from organ failure. This, I am told is the hardest way to go. Of course, the Scarecrow's death may be the most desirable. He will probably die in his sleep still easing on down the road.

Chapter 5
THE WHERE

Fact:
There are three places to die

Where would you like to die? Most people might answer "In my sleep." Sleeping is more a state of being, rather than a geographic location. For every other memorable moment in your life you have answered the question, "Where?" For my wedding, I want to get married naked on a beach in Mexico adorned with a single corsage. For my 50th birthday, I will hike the Grand Canyon blindfolded. For the birth of my son, I will be in the shallow waters of Lake Tahoe. When thinking about the location to celebrate our milestones the imagination is unstoppable. With death, it stops here. In deciding where to die, you have four options but only three choices. You can choose to die at home, at a hospice center, or in a hospital. Sudden death is by nature unforeseeable (although the *Tibetan Book of the Dead*, states there are warning signs prior to sudden death - dreams, animal totems and warnings from loved ones.) The fourth option is that you can die anywhere suddenly or if you stay any place long enough you will die in that location, which like paying taxes, is a loose definition of Choice.

Terminal illness comes with the advantage of better accuracy of days left to live. Dying is only a part of living and hopefully that part comes after 80 or 90 years. Elderly people feel lucky to have a home death. Just as home births shed its label as an archaic village practice to a holistic choice, home deaths are still a sacred option that can be planned and executed well. My dearest aunt laid in the bed next to her father while he was dying. She was his eldest child, primary caretaker and a physician. She described his last moments as "wonderful." He was at home in his comfortable bed wearing flannel pajamas and enjoying a fresh Caribbean breeze. Control is what dying at home allows. Choosing to die at home with the right preparation, honest dialogue, and minor medical knowledge ensures everyone is attending the same party. Your sons, your daughters, and your loved ones understand the point of your little get together. You, the guest of honor, are dying. Understanding this simple fact is crucial because your loved ones may have the urge to do something. They may feel scared as your face becomes contorted with real or imagined pain. Give your family permission to sit calmly, breathe, weep, and possibly pray.

However, everything isn't for everybody. Families may not be comfortable handling a dead body at home. You, the dying, may also opt out because of the added security of having a medical professional present just in case. There may be children in the house that are too young to witness a dying person. More commonly though, is that no one recognizes that you are dying. A sudden change in your condition may have occurred which causes concern. Your family members panic. You are whisked away to the hospital or hospice center.

Hospice is basically the birthing center version for the dying. The comfort and coziness of a home-like setting with the added plus of intravenous injections for pain, oxygen for breathlessness, and the just-in-case medical professional. Doctors cannot admit just anybody to a hospice center. Someone arbitrarily defined six months left to live as the cut-off to be eligible for hospice care. Fortunately, not just terminally ill cancer patients can die in a hospice center. Patients with organ failure and frailty are also accepted. My paternal aunt died in a hospice center in Florida after being parasitized with ovarian cancer. Her pastor played the clarinet and her younger sister held her hand until the end.

Modern medicine has made dying in a hospital less than comfortable. There is the incessant beeping of various machines which range from cellphones to the characteristic cardiac chime of beep-silence-beep-silence-beep-silence. Glaring fluorescent lights are ubiquitous. Added to this, the annoying pleasant chatter of people at their day jobs. "Excuse me," you manage a whisper from your death bed in the intensive care unit, "I am dying. Do you think Aunty Emma's new chili recipe can wait?"

For many dying, in a hospital is not intentional. People with organ failure arrive by the busloads to the ambulance bay of the hospital. They have had an acute episode which exacerbated their underlying chronic illness. Western medicine is good at treating emergencies, quick fixes of all types. There are machines to assist breathing after your lungs have failed. There are drugs to lower your potassium reversing the efforts of failing kidneys. The healthcare team is privileged to have skills which help the sick and diseased live longer, which is not the same as helping the dying live longer. The distinction between the two is hardly obvious.

It is not always possible to make the sick better in the hospital. This is humbling to medical professionals. Doctors, along with the medical team, may be unsuccessful. This may be not as much their fault but your choice. You are choosing to die in a hospital if this is your fourth admission for an acute problem within six months. Multiple intubations for poorly controlled asthma is a sure fire way to die in a hospital. Your high-fat-no-excercise-lifestyle once more blocks the stents in your heart so off you go to the emergency department. Whether you realize it or not you are making a decision to die in a hospital.

When you die in an emergency department, expect lots of strangers to touch you. A nurse may repeatedly poke your arm with a needle. The patient care technician may insert a temperature probe rectally. Expect also noise. Not only from machines, but also the drunk patient who happens to be seven months pregnant and screaming "Barack Obama is my daddy!" while beating her chest clothed in a dirty white tank top and imitating a forest gorilla. This person could be your neighboring patient or their visiting relative that you could reach out a hand and touch. Then there is the noise of medical speak. The loud murmurings of the doctor to the nurses; the nurses to the patient care technician; or the all powerful desk clerk declaring in the intercom overhead "All visitors out!" These cast of characters are all party-crashers to your final moments. If you are dying, this may be no big deal and you may not care. However, your family members might have a need for quietude. Their grieving now becomes a public spectacle. Reciting scriptures in your ear as you die is less than intimate.

Some hospitals can't afford to have a designated grievance room. In most inner city or community emergency departments, every square footage is prime real estate.

Bereavement rooms don't make the cut. These exist more commonly on other medical floors, and almost always in the ICU.

Dying in other parts of the hospital is much the same as dying in the emergency department. The disturbing noise, the weird character of strangers, and the light intensity are only slightly varied.

Visitors and employees do pause for the dead in a hospital. Hugs are offered by the staff. Boxes of tissues are made available. It is still a moment of significance. After a brief reprieve other strangers will introduce themselves to your family. They will inquire about organ donation, autopsy, and funeral pick-up times from the morgue.

Make a deliberate choice of where you want to die not a happenstance mistake. Choose a place whether it be in a home, a hospice center, or a hospital. Choosing to die in a hospital does not mean your dying cannot be infused with religion. The Iman can pray with you. The Orthodox Jews require any clothes that the deceased blood touched is to be buried with them. In keeping with this custom, doctors have disrobed and relinquished their blood stained scrub pants. Hindus require the body not to be moved until after the Pandit has recited the final truism. Different cultures are allowed to perform the last rites of passage as they see fit. Now the party is finally over for you.

Fairytale:
Oh, the places you can die!

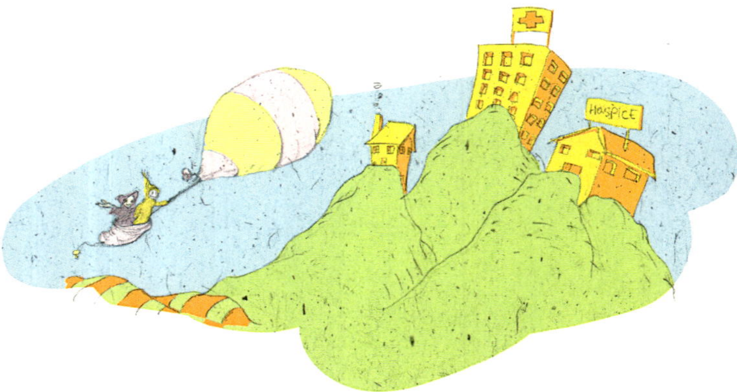

Congratulations!
Today is your day.
You're off to great places.
You're off and away!

Where do you want it to happen?
Where do you want it to be?
When it comes to deciding
where to die,
Your choices are four
but really only three.

You're on your own.

And you know what you know.
You can die at the hospital,
hospice or home.
The fourth option
is not much of a choice.
Like lightning striking you
on your porch
Falling under an avalanche
or a kick from a horse.

This of course means
you can die anywhere.
So look up the block
and down the streets.
Look 'em over with care.
You might say,
"I choose not to go there."

Dying at home
is the best I should think.
Your loved ones are there.
Sharing a drink.
In the living room or bedroom

With a blanket and a pillow
In your favorite color pink.

But everything ain't for everybody
So off to the hospital you go
Before your atoms shatter
and you become antimatter.
Expect lights, beeps, burps and chatter
As things start to happen.
Don't worry. Don't sigh.
Oh! The Places You Can Die!

You may choose a hospice
to end the good fight.
Oxygen is there and morphine for pain.
Trained professionals
led by the whole gang.

Dying in an emergency department
I am sorry to say
Strangers will touch you
In every kind of way
The nurse will poke you

The doctor may cut open your chest
Prepare for a rectal probe
when you should be at rest.

Expect a clerk to announce
"All visitors out!"
The moan of the sick
and tired of waiting
The moan of impatience
and those like you fading.

You may not care
But your family might
Grieving publicly
while reading your dying rites.

Once you've started in one place
It will be much too hard to escape
So choose
Choose carefully.

Oh! The Places You Can Die!

On you will go
though the pain be great
On you will go
though your breathing be late.

Be your name Keisha, Seema
or Johnson Jay
You're off to great places
So get on your way.

Oh! The Places You Can Die!

Chapter 6
THE WHO

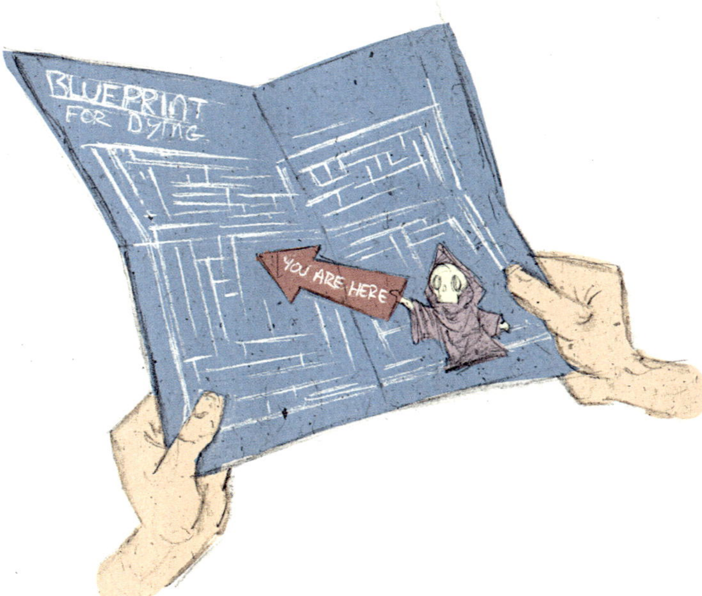

Fact:
There is a blueprint for dying

It is a well known fact that all who are born die. However, because of abortion and miscarriage not all who are alive are born and so the dead outnumber the living. Given how common dying is, there is a surprising dearth of information and scientific research on the actual process of dying.

We know with week to week precision, the process of a growing fetus until it is born, and yet we know very little about the stages of dying. It is a process which can take place in seconds or hours depending on if one dies suddenly or not. Even the writings on near-death experience by definition miss the physical symptoms that are common to all dying creatures. Much of the Western literature on dying is from hospice providers. On the other hand, in Eastern literature there are volumes of writings dedicated to death and dying.

The Tibetans have a monopoly on the discourse of dying. Their books should be a required reading in medical school. When the most famous book to come out of a country is entitled *The Tibetan Book of the Dead* several scholars have put much thought into the topic. The Tibetans recommend dying in the *sleeping lion pose*. A person should lie on their right side, left hand on the left thigh, right hand under the chin closing the right nostril. Such advice is as straightforward as the Good Witch Glenda telling Dorothy click your heels three times preferably in some red pumps while chanting, "There's no place like home."

The Tibetans describe an outer body dissolving and an inner mind/consciousness dissolution at the time of death. The five steps of the outer body dissolving are common to all living creatures. The inner dissolution relies on one's belief that the body is separate from the mind. There is a basic Eastern belief that the mind houses the consciousness, and at the time of death, the consciousness continues to exist. For many Westerners of Christian, Muslim, and Jewish faiths, this assumption may not be true. This chapter is not intended to be a Buddhism-lite discourse, so only the physical shedding of the body will be discussed.

The five stages of dying occur after the acceptance of death, which has already been elucidated in chapter one, by Little Red Riding Hood.

In the first stage of dying the senses fade. One can identify sounds of people talking but not the words. Anyone who has ever fallen into a drunken stupor can relate to the phenomenon where language fades from specific words to high and low pitched sounds. The melody of the music is there but the words have withered. One can see objects in front of you but not recognize any details. It is sort of like driving in a blizzard. Similarly, the senses of smell, touch, and taste fade away. After the senses all fade away, the second phase is over.

In the second phase the body loses all its strength. One has no power to sit upright or hold one's head up. Hollywood has over-fed us images of the dying hero or heroine. The wounded soldier is lying in the clutches of his beloved. He utters his final words staring into her eyes, collapsing amidst loud sobs. This role is not hard to imagine. Restlessness may ensue. Narcotics provided for this type of psychic pain may be helpful. Some texts say one feels as though one is falling, sinking underground, or being crushed by a great weight. One's complexion fades, and becomes pale. It becomes harder to open one's eyes.

In the third phase, one loses control of all bodily fluids. The nose and eyes run. One becomes incontinent. The lips are drawn and bloodless, the mouth is sticky and one becomes thirsty. Bodily sensations dwindle and alternate between pain and pleasure.

Initially saliva may accumulate in one's mouth giving rise to the death rattle, the noise emitted as the ability to swallow is lost but breathing continues. Loved ones often misinterpret this noise as evidence of "the agony of death." Suctioning the saliva is an option. However, this may ease one's families discomfort but probably does not help or hinder your passage. Progression to this third phase means that you have rung the doorbell of Death, you stand on the welcome mat and listen to the creak of the door as it opens.

In the fourth stage of dying, all warmth leaves the body zooming in from feet and hands towards the heart. One can no longer drink or digest anything. The mind swings between clarity and confusion. It is more difficult to perceive anything with lucidity.

Dying has become highly medicalized. Modern medicine has created many tricks to alter these stages. No one really knows if these interventions assist or impede the dying process. Morphine and its ilk like fentanyl and propofol can help decrease restlessness and psychic pain. Patients with terminal illness often endure severe pain therefore judicious use of narcotics is encouraged. Intravenous fluids or water may relieve thirst. Victims dying from organ failure have breathlessness and air hunger. The use of oxygen is advantageous for these patients. The decision whether or not to have pain medicine, oxygen, or water should be declared in your dying plan.

The final stage of dying has to do with breathing. Life begins and ends with a breath. In this fifth stage it becomes harder to breathe. The in-breaths are short and choppy. The out-breaths are longer. One may be gasping for air. Western medicine defines this as agonal breathing and is a sign of imminent death. Your last contact with the physical environment is slipping away. All vital signs are gone. One is certifiable dead according to modern medicine. Congratulations! You made it.

Fairytale:
Five Little Piggys

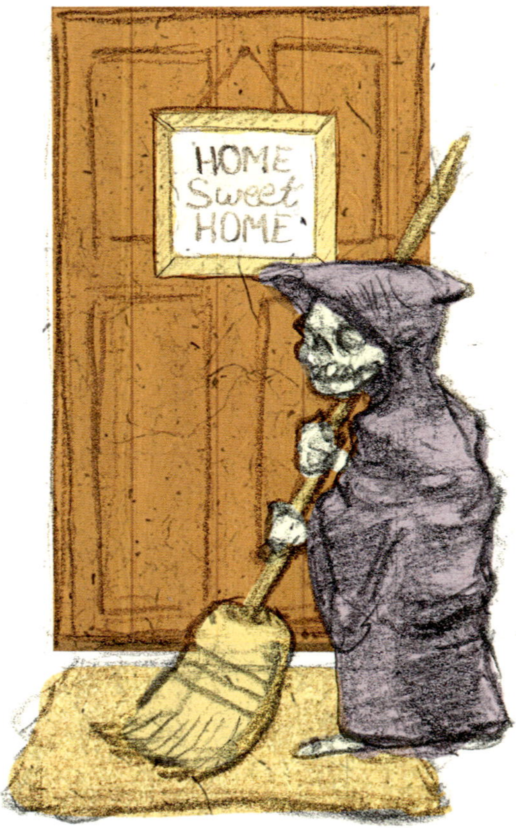

A long time ago there were five pigs. These were the first famous Piggys. Before the big bad blowing Wolf, there was a little biped porcine. You may recall, that this little piggy went to the market. It was more than a place to buy food, the North Africans refer to this meeting place as the Souk. He went to buy a few things for his brothers.

They were not well. This is putting it mildly because they were actually, all five of them, dying. The first piggy strolled past the green limes, the barrel of yellow tumeric, and the rows of red tomatoes. His head turned as a woman yelled, "Fresh fish! Fresh fish! Five dollars!" Piggy almost stepped on a mangy dog barking at a young girl. She was dangling a blue ball in front of the dog's face. An extra finger was on her left hand. The rankness of the fish mixed with a wisp of jasmine made the pig wince. Having purchased all the items on his list, he started the journey back to his brothers.

There was a wide meadow of grass between the market and his tiny home. Every few steps he took towards his family, he looked back to find the little girl with the ball. She grew smaller and smaller until he had almost reached his door and all that remained of her was a black dot. The din from the market was all he could make out. All the wonderful sights, smells, and sounds faded. This stage of dying is now complete.

The true beginning phase of dying is the acceptance that death is possible and inevitable. Poor little piggy missed this stage of dying because, unlike you, he was a simpleton.

The second piggy stayed home. He was tired and listless. He could not sit up. He laid in bed waiting for his brother to return from the market. "Silly little fool", he thought, "What is taking him so long? I am dying here. You promised me a foot rub with sandalwood oil." The second piggy's skin grew pale. He could hardly open his eyes. Later he would recall as his body lost all its strength that he was falling, sinking underground, or being crushed by a great weight. As he finished the second stage of dying, he started to fidget in bed. This was quite annoying to the other piggys.

The third piggy had roast beef. It was the fulfillment of a dying wish. He should have had a glass of water. His mouth felt sticky and he was thirsty. His eyes and nose were running. He peed on himself. He too was waiting for his wayward brother to hurry home from the market. As he alternated between pain and pleasure, he wondered what could be taking Brother Piggy so long. His brother knew the way to the market and was bringing back poppy seeds for pain. The third pig's lips became drawn and bloodless. Saliva pooled in his mouth. He could no longer swallow. He began the death rattle. During this third phase of dying, he circled the drain of the kitchen sink belonging to Death.

The fourth piggy had none. He could not drink or digest anything. Plus he was chilly. All the warmth left his body. First his feet then his hands. His heart was the last thing to stay warm. He also fleetingly remembered his brother had gone somewhere. He had forgotten why.

The last little piggy huffed and puffed as he gasped for air. Pigs like humans begin life with an inhale and end with an exhale. Poor piggy's eyes rolled up into his head. The legendary adventure concludes as always: He went wee wee wee all the way home.

Chapter 7
The Immortal Dilemma

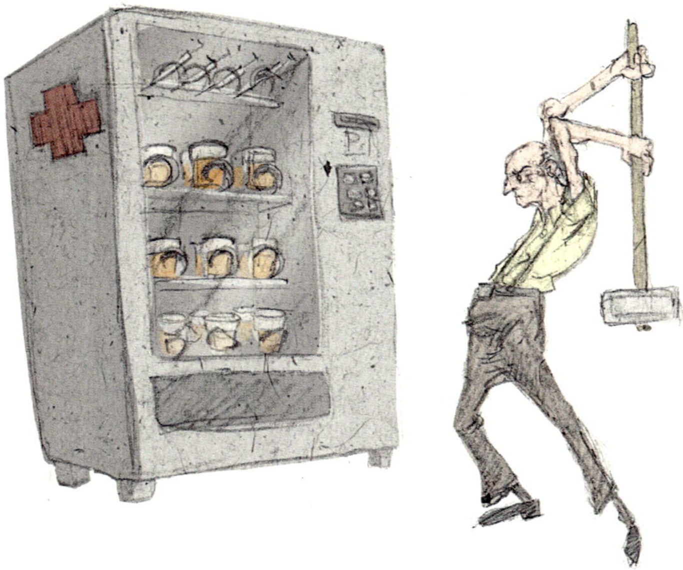

Fact:
Dying can be planned or not planned

The immortal dilemma is a set of four questions that each human being will have to answer, willingly or not. Even silence is an answer. Why leave the plan of your final moments to chance. Let it be an occasion of celebration. Invite the guests. Choose the music and a few of your favorite things. Or you may decide you want solitude. At least you have made a choice. Your family and loved ones will cherish this decision just as well.

As you solve your immortal dilemma keep in mind the following:

1. Know Your Options

Where do you want to die?

If you are dying at home, you will have much more control than if you are dying in a hospital-like setting. For example, dimmed lights are not an option in the emergency department but might be in a hospice.

2. Examine Your Feelings

How do you feel about your own dying and death? For many it is uncomfortable and strange, to think about their own death. It may be downright terrifying for loved ones to think about your death. You are planning for dying which is a natural and unavoidable stage of life. Discuss your feelings with your family, caregivers, and medical professionals.

3. Consider Your Priorities

What is important to you and your loved ones as you are dying? If you are part of a tight devotional community, then maybe having your religious leader present is a top priority. Decide what is important and make the necessary arrangements.

4. Meet With Your Medical Professional

The focus of the medical community is to prolong life. This is often at the detriment of the aged and feeble. Many health professionals feel like they have failed if their patient dies. Being open to a conversation about dying, makes it easier for you and your caregivers to understand when the stage of dying begins. Discuss your dying plan to ensure that everyone is in agreement of how it will be executed. Help them to help you.

Immortal Dilemma

Complete. Save. Share.

1. Location:

Where do you want to die?

( ) home

( ) hospice

( ) hospital

2. Attendants:

Who do you want present?

I would like my:

( ) partner

( ) parents/elders

( ) religious figure

( ) siblings

( ) friends

( ) children

( ) pet

( ) ______________

3. Amenities:

What would you like?

I would like:

( ) music

( ) soft lighting

( ) my favorite___________

( )as few interruptions as possible

( ) my mouth moistened

( ) IV fluids

( ) ___________________

4. Pain Relief:

What kind of pain relief do you want?

I would like:

( ) acupuncture

( ) meditation

( ) breathing techniques

( ) prayer

( ) standard narcotics

( ) whatever is suggested

( ) nothing

Fairytale:
So long Winnie-the-Pooh

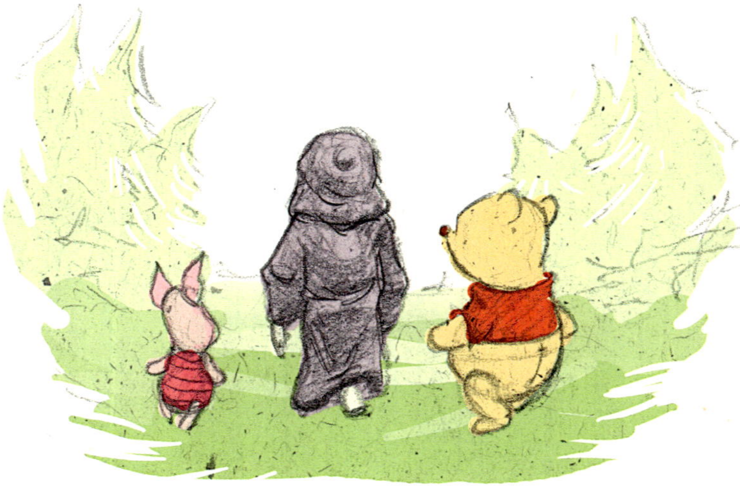

Begin dictation:
This is Dr. Owl.
Medical Record: 520052
Patient Name: Edward Bear aka
Winnie-the-Pooh
Date of Birth: January 18, 1915

Winne-the-Pooh is a 98 year-old brown bear who has an insatiable craving for honey and all things sweet. Unsurprisingly, this addiction led to a terrible case of uncontrolled diabetes. Despite stoutness exercises, alternative sweeteners, and even a few home remedies, his kidneys ultimately failed.

Two years ago, the patient was started on hemodialysis. The trip from the forest edge to the dialysis center was cumbersome and lengthy. One week ago, Mr. Pooh chose to forego any further cleansing of his blood and expressed his wish to die under his favorite oak tree with his friends, Rabbit, Piglet, and of course Christopher Robin. Pooh who knows everything about everything has made it explicit that there are to be no overzealous medical interventions at the time of his dying. He will allow a natural death. All documents have been signed indicating that he is not a full code and there will be no attempts at resuscitation.

Piglet, his best friend and primary caretaker, has expressed concern that he does not want Pooh to die too early. On the other hand, dying too late is equally as undesirable.

I have explained that in the end everything will be alright. If it's not alright then it's not the end. And the line between prolonging life versus expediting dying lies squarely upon the breath. No effort will be made to assist his breathing. He will die naturally.

As a scientist, I wish all my patients could understand that water gets you wet and life makes you die. I have asked Pooh to make a list. The first item is a bed of soft leaves. He has asked Rabbit, as an expert in foraging and an aficionado of all things soft, to be the chief executor of item number one. Rabbit understands the monumental task ahead of him. After years of ingesting the byproduct of bees copulating with flowers, the girth of Pooh Bear is no less than gargantuan.

Pooh has repeatedly conveyed his anxiety about pain. Specifically, there is to be none. Pooh disagrees with my advice on pain relief. As it is impolite to contradict a dying bear, I have obliged his second request. Piglet has gathered jars, cups, even syringes filled with honey for psychic pain, breathing pain, and break-through pain.

The final request of Mr. Bear is for Christopher Robin to sing Pooh's prized song:

"Row, row, row your boat.
Gently down the stream.
Merrily, merrily, merrily, merrily
Life is but a dream."

Initially, this plantigrade mammal had a third request to spend his final moments in an actually raft. I expended a generous amount of time elucidating the metaphor: the boat refers to one's self and rowing is an arduous practice that takes perfection, but also directs the vessel. When sung as a group, the act of rowing becomes a unifier, as oars should be in sync for the progression of a rowboat. The idea that we travel along a certain stream, which is yet another metaphor for time, and this stream suggests boundaries in the path of choices and our free will to eat honey. The third line prescribes that challenges should be greeted not only with joy but without the worry of future problems. The final line, *"Life is but a dream,"* is perhaps the most meaningful. Life may be regarded as having a comparable significance as that of a dream, such that troubles, and dying should rightly be placed in this category of inconveniences, are seen in the context of a lesser reality once one has awakened.

Forgive me, dear reader, for wasting your time stating the obvious about this nursery rhyme. One can never tell the difference between palpable and common, especially by persons that study and believe things written by an owl claiming to be a doctor of medicine.

My entire explanation proved too difficult for the patient to grasp. Upon acknowledging that honey on a boat might spill, the idea was quickly abandoned as absurd.

Having lived a long life filled with close friends and in keeping with his habit, lots of honey, Pooh has given instructions for his dying party. Crying is allowed and even encouraged. Tissue boxes embossed with "Farewell Winnie-the-Pooh" will be made available. Wailing is not permitted. Screaming, screeching, and other irritating sounds will result in an immediate eviction from the party.

My presence, as a feathered creature, whose natural call is a perpetual question, is an exception. *Who? Who?* Piglet assures me, *we know who, Pooh is who, Winnie-the-Pooh.* Upon hearing his name, Pooh gazes at each one of his friends - Rabbit, Christopher Robin, myself, and finally Piglet. His last words:

The hardest part is what to leave behind...
It's time to let go!

License number 372882.
Dictation complete.

Chapter Eight
The Art of Dying

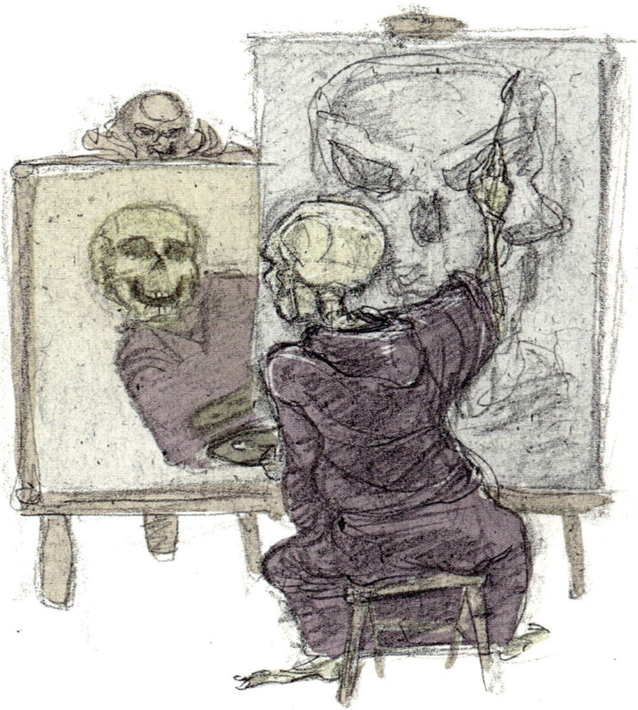

It is difficult to extricate dying from spirituality. For most of the world, it is impossible and undesirable. People of all faiths believe dying is a journey "home" to meet their maker. Religious and spiritual texts of all creeds agree on two things. At the moment of death, it is best to die among soothing sounds, pleasant smells, and soft light. Life is best lived in comfort. So it follows that to die in coziness is a natal right. The choice between dying on Egyptian cotton spread over a king bed with your son singing "Amazing Grace" versus dying on a hospital gurney under blaring fluorescent lights, is obvious. Secondly, dying is not the time for pettiness. Forget the twenty dollars your neighbor owes you. Encounter only love at the moment of dying.

Plan your last hours as you would a graduation ceremony, a birthday party, or a vacation. Where do you want to die? Instead of a hospital machine alarming, you could listen to Chopin or Bob Marley. Who do you want present? Perhaps your beloved repeating a favorite Rumi verse. What will make you the most comfortable - your hands massaged by your granddaughter or snuggling up with your favorite pillow. Possibly, you may want to be alone. This too is an alternative decision. Your last moments are absolutely personal. It is your creative experience which is not repeatable nor transmissible to another person.

Dying is so important to death that one must rehearse it. Athletes do not start preparing on the day of the race. Practice controlling the breath and the emotions as a foundation for the dying process. When medicine can no longer help the disease process, it is time to optimize placebo, faith, diet, and spiritual practice. The goal is for all parties to agree that when dying has begun - the objective is a peaceful death. These are the elements of a good death which is still possible.

The memory of your last moments will remain with your loved ones for the rest of their lives. The ability to give and receive words should be maintained until the end. The words of the dying carry meaning, prophecy, good wishes, or even an ill omen. Who can forget the last curse of the melting Wicked Witch of the West: "This is not over, I'll get you my pretty!" A more memorable ending was made by a friend's mother who after all of her children had gathered around her hospital bed, she looked out the window and whispered, "All's well that ends well."

Dying is life's greatest mystery. Possessions you have accumulated will remain. Time is the only thing that runs out. It is the most precious gift. The secret to a good life and a good death is to experience each minute as if an eternity lives in it. The world needs you to believe that your every deed matters. Your every word matters more than you can imagine. Imagine this moment as the one you lived your life to get to. It is.

About the Author

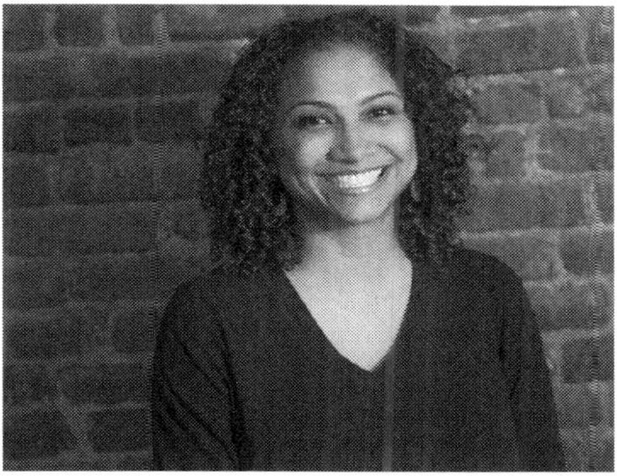

Placid Bone, M.D. combines the best of Eastern medicine and Western science. *Mortality & Magic: Facts & Fairytales for the Hereafter*, weaves together proven medical insight with parodies of classic fairytales into a humorous guide on the ups and downs of death and dying. It is a good book on dying well.

While becoming a board certified physician, Dr. Bone studied mortality around the world, and received a medical degree from New York University, and emergency medicine training at Harvard and Yale. Her publications include *Emergency Clinics of North America: Oncologic Emergencies* and *EP Monthly: An*

Introduction to Palliative Care. Placid is a developer and facilitator of seminars in Education in Palliative and End-of-Life Care for Emergency Medicine (EPEC-EM).

She has worked in both academic and community medical settings throughout the Northeastern United States, as well as in India, South Africa, Cuba, Guyana, and the United Arab Emirates among others. Placid has studied Ayurvedic Medicine, India's oldest healing system, at the University of Pune and at the Arsha Vaidya in Coimbatore, India.

Placid lives in Brooklyn, NY with three boys who claim to be her offspring, and a poet who is the alleged donor of their extraordinary genetic code.

Dr. Bone has attended countless dying moments with her patients. This is not a slight on her medical expertise, but a testament that every day death is near and especially so in the emergency department.

Disclaimer

This book is designed to provide accurate information on the subject of dying. Names and situations have been altered to protect each creature's privacy. The author is not offering any medical services by the publication of this bock. As each situation is unique, questions specific to your individual case should be addressed by the appropriate professional (or God) to ensure careful evaluation.

The author and publisher disclaim any liability or loss incurred as a consequence of the use cr application of the contents of this work.

Please feel free to write a review, before or after you die, if the information provided proves valuable to you and your loved ones in any way at all: placidbone@gmail.com.

Immortal Dilemma

Complete. Save. Share.

1. Location:

Where do you want to die?

( ) home
( ) hospice
( ) hospital

2. Attendants:

Who do you want present?

I would like my:

( ) partner
( ) parents/elders
( ) religious figure
( ) siblings
( ) friends
( ) children
( ) pet
( ) ______________

3. Amenities:

What would you like?

I would like:

( ) music

( ) soft lighting

( ) my favorite____________

( ) as few interruptions as possible

( ) my mouth moistened

( ) IV fluids

( ) ____________________

4. Pain Relief:

What kind of pain relief do you want?

I would like:

( ) acupuncture

( ) meditation

( ) breathing techniques

( ) prayer

( ) standard narcotics

( ) whatever is suggested

( ) nothing

STORY
OF MY
LIFE